What you see is not how I feel

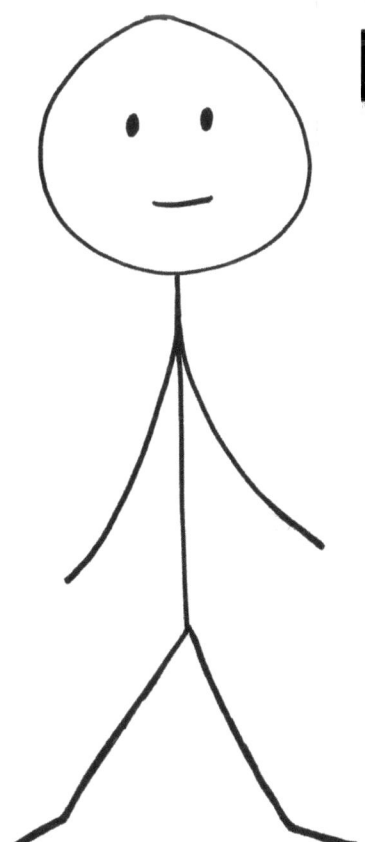

Myalgic Encephalomyelitis
(ME/CFS)

Anderson

www.whatyouseebooks.wordpress.com

Revised Version

Written from the heart for all who struggle with ME or other "invisible" chronic illnesses.

Myalgic Encephalomyelitis (ME)
Chronic Fatigue Syndrome (CFS)
Systemic Exertion Intolerance Disease (SEID)

What you see is not how I feel
Copyright © 2021 by Anderson

Rev. date: 03-03-2020

All rights reserved. No part of this publication may be reproduced, distributed, or transmitted in any form or by any means, including photocopying, recording, or other electronic or mechanical methods, without the prior written permission of the author, except in the case of brief quotations embodied in critical reviews and certain other non-commercial uses permitted by copyright law.

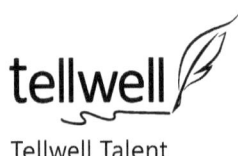

Tellwell Talent
www.tellwell.ca

ISBN
978-0-2288-1970-7 (Hardcover)
978-0-2288-1968-4 (Paperback)
978-0-2288-1969-1 (eBook)

This book includes most of my symptoms of Myalgic Encephalomyelitis over the last five years. Not everyone has all or the same symptoms. It is not intended to set expectations going forward, but to simply present what it is like living with my intensity of ME.

With deep appreciation for Dr. A.L. Sayao, BSc, MD, FRCPC, Neurologist, UBC MS Hospital - the first and only doctor until diagnosis that recognized that it might be ME. Invaluable advice: go home, start doing yoga and see a psychologist – you need to talk.

With the deepest of thanks to E. Dicasmirro, Trauma and Somatic Psychotherapist, RPT, CBC — who listened professionally but "warmly" in kindness and compassion without judgment, helping me take the first steps to recovery of my mind and body.

Thank you Dr. R. Arseneau, MD, FRCPC, MA(Ed), MBA, FACP, CGP, Internist – diagnosing doctor who knew immediately, and the understanding staff at the Complex Chronic Diseases Program, BC Women's Hospital, 2016-2018.

Dr. P. Kryskow, MD, CCFP, Pain Specialist, MuscleMD clinic - your inspiring insights, example and wisdom are as powerful as the needles -Thank you, thank you.

Ongoing appreciation to Dr. Benetiz-Gomez, MD — who has seen me through this whole experience.

What you see is not how I feel

I don't look sick or even all that tired.

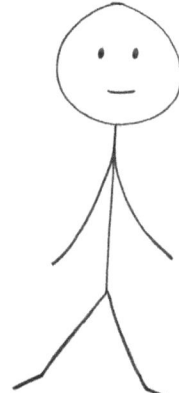

When you see this

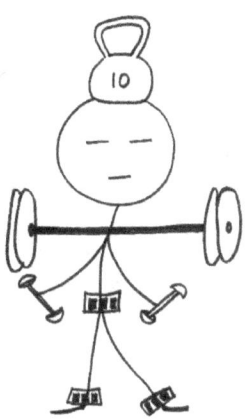

I feel like this

This is how I always feel.

I could just give up, atrophy, and never try to keep going, or I could just live in spite of it.

When I keep going

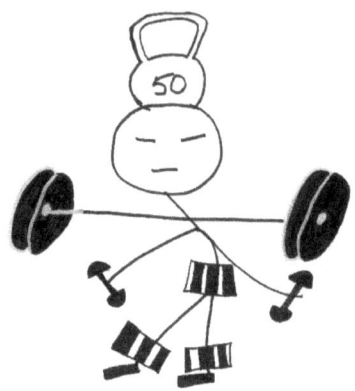

the weights get heavier and heavier

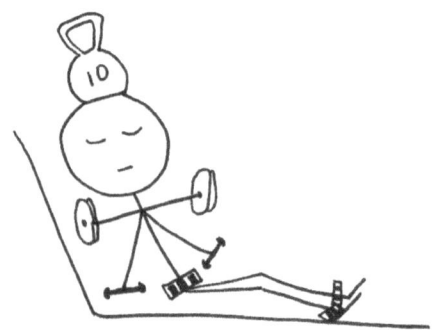

Rest or sleep only makes the weights lighter again

I can't just put them down. They are always there.

I always hear ringing in my ears.

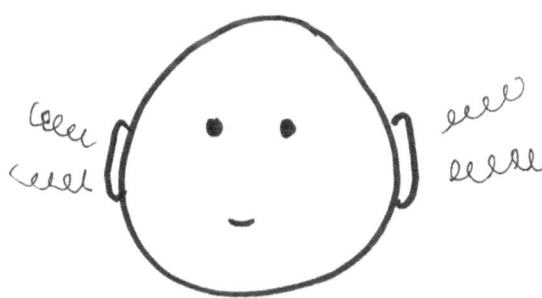

When I keep going the ringing gets louder and louder, until it is such a distraction (along with the heavier weights) that it affects my thinking.

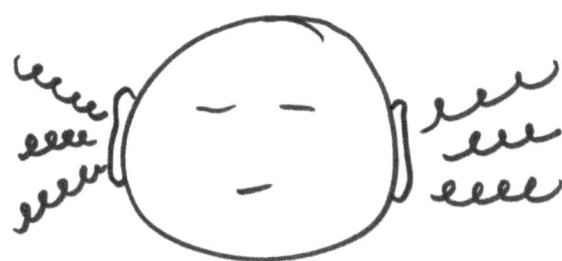

Then small things are overwhelming. Decisions and reasoning are difficult. Stress compounds all of this.

I just want to go hide.

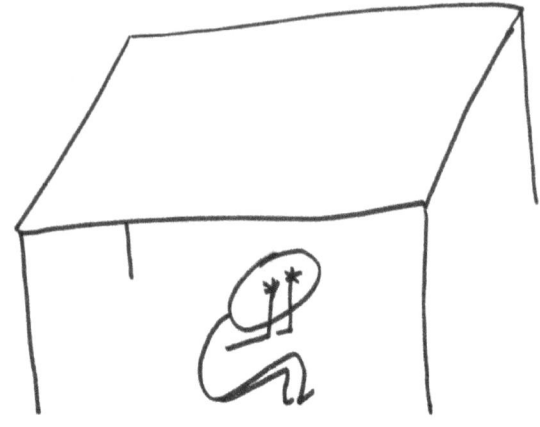

and sometimes cry

I get random zapping pains in my muscles and joints, and even on my skin.

Sometimes, the pains are quick and shocking. Other times, they recur rapidly in seconds, minutes, hours, days, or weeks.

Some pains never go away — like in my jaws. These pains zap into my eardrums.

I press them hard till the pain stops

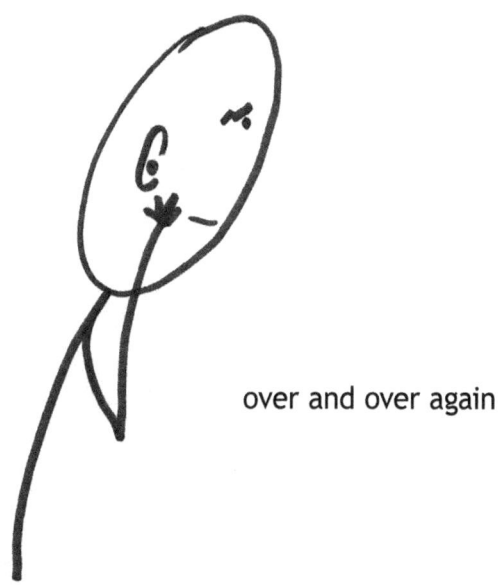

over and over again

Stress makes me clench my jaw — making the pain worse.

My feet always tingle and burn — day and night. Stress makes the tingling and burning go up my legs as high as my thighs. I get the sensation of tight bands around my ankles.

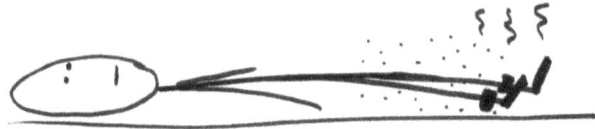

I feel it all more at night when my feet burn hotter

    the tingling is stronger

        and the bands are tighter

I flip the covers on and off — this doesn't help my sleep.

    You see this, if you see me

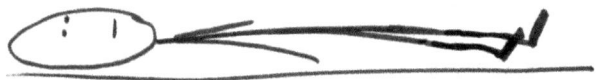

    only the outside

Yoga is one thing my doctors tell me to do.

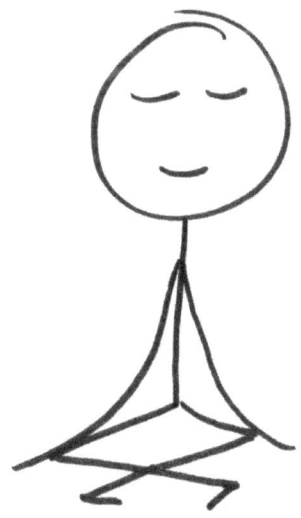

It is expensive
but for me it is not a luxury
It is a lifeline

Yoga strengthens muscles while not using too much energy. It calms the mind and central nervous system. Yoga reduces stress – allowing the body to do what it does naturally, heal.

At yoga, you see this

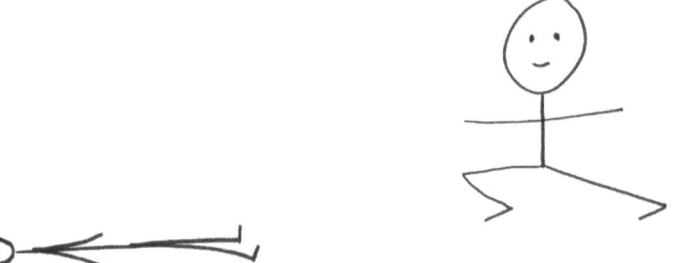

I feel like this

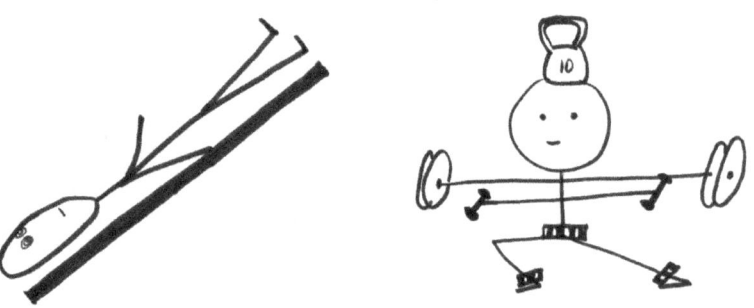

Pressure builds in my head.
The weights push down.
The floor tilts or moves in waves — sometimes both.

I am always dizzy with a constant sense of movement. I can never get off the boat.

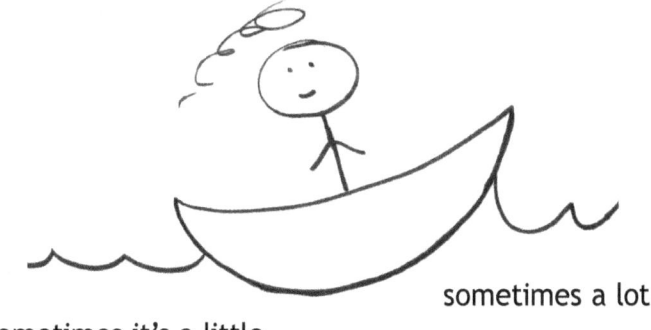

Sometimes it's a little   sometimes a lot

When I can turn quickly, I look like this

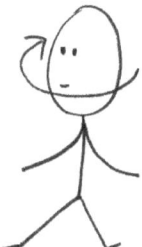

Other times it feels like my head is swinging with outward force with the weight on top.

I feel like this

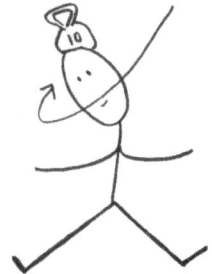

I never know what I will feel,
like I'm spinning or I simply turned.
All you see is that I turned.

Many symptoms I have to tell you about as they are happening, but I don't — you would think I was nuts.

Nausea comes on randomly and can last an hour, a day, a week, or a month.

I look like this

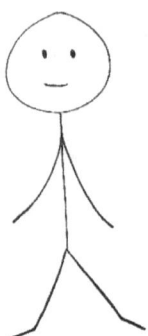

I feel like this

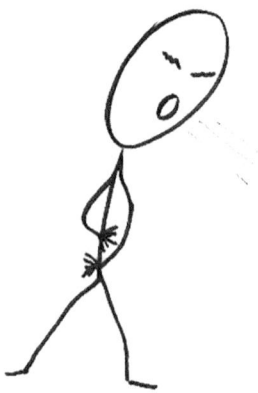

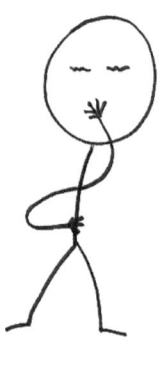

Some people with ME regularly throw up.

When I sit at the computer for more than 30 minutes,

You see this

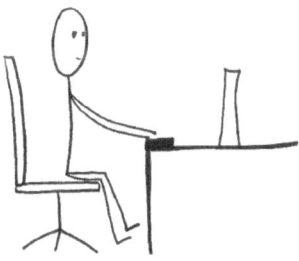

I start feeling like the desk, the chair and I, are tilting like this

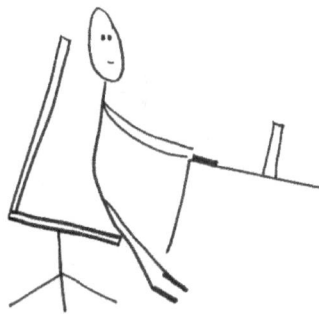

I start leaning and pressing backward so I don't fall forward. I really won't, but it is disconcerting.

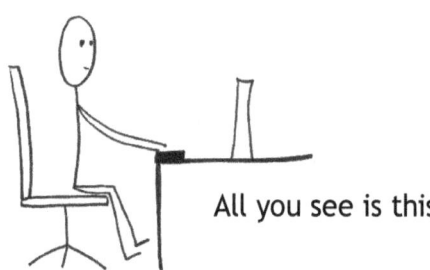

All you see is this

In a restaurant you see this.

Then you see this

My head feels heavier and heavier

My ears start ringing louder, social weariness sets in, and my brain starts to scramble

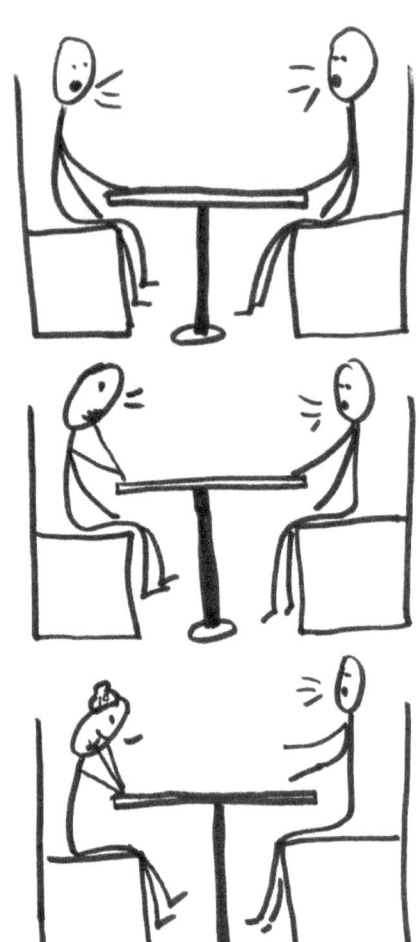

What you see is not how I feel

I quickly get Sensory Overload.

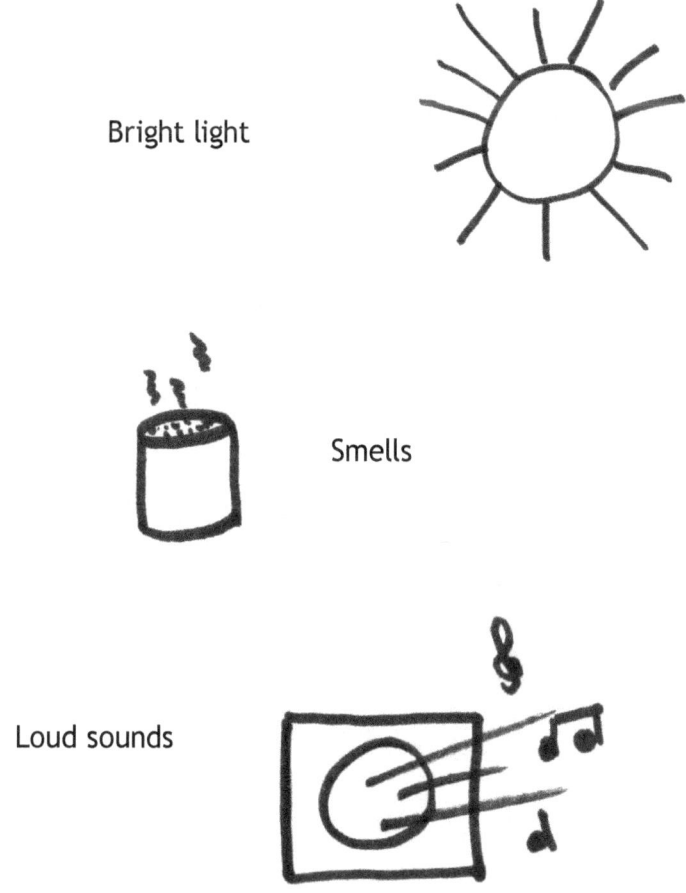

These are overpowering and overwhelming.

Sometimes I simply get tired of coping, but life is worth living even though I manage differently now. I plan my days and try to choose which activities I do — when, where, and how long. I plan my rest and sleep times.

I get really frustrated when it takes so long to do what I used to do quickly, or don't get to complete it because I have run out of steam.

Finally, I simply accept that it was all I could do "today" and try to be glad for what I did get started or finished.

I often feel like I have the flu. When I get the real flu, I can't really tell the difference.

I regularly have a sore throat. It can be dull or really sore.

It stings when I pee.

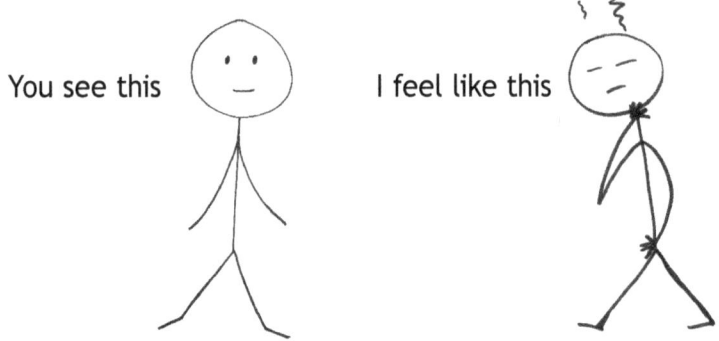

Symptoms always worsen the more I push on, the more tired I get, and the more stress I have.

I start walking into door jams hitting my shoulder. I get clumsy, dropping and spilling things. I cut and burn myself, and miss the counter when I mean to put a dish on it.

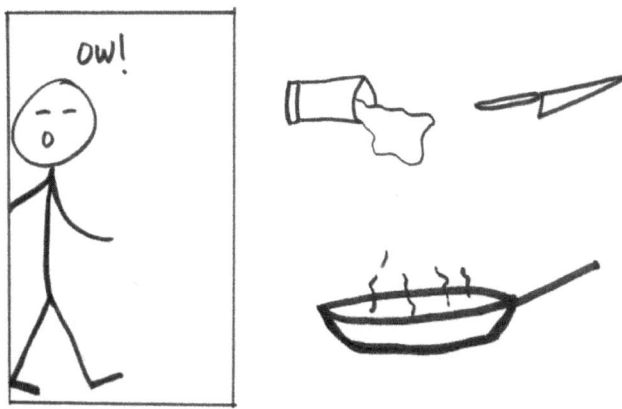

I struggle to find the right words. My mouth stiffens and some sounds are hard to form.

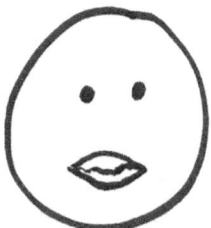

My body *can* do physical activities. My muscles do have strength, but only till the energy is spent.

People only see this

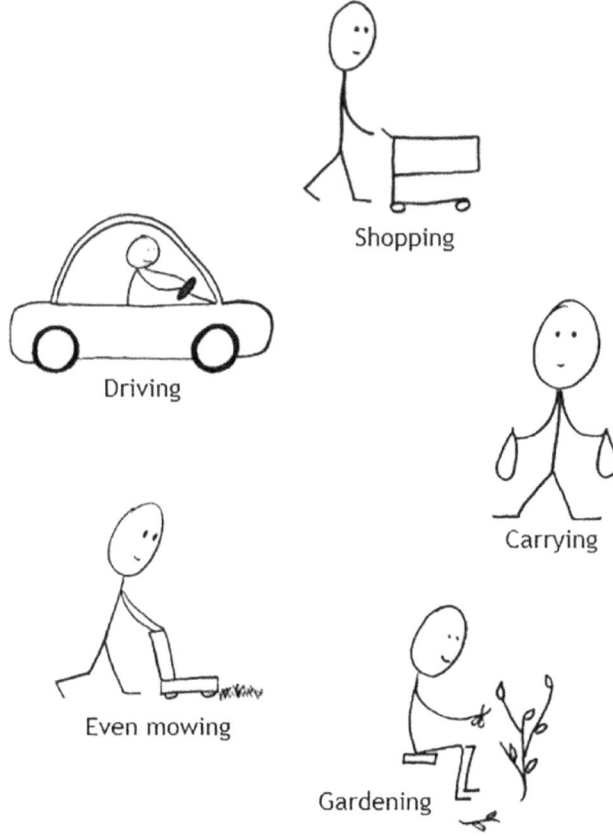

Shopping

Driving

Carrying

Even mowing

Gardening

Life happens — these things are necessary and then necessary again. I'm lucky I can do them.

What you see is not how I feel

What people don't see is the cost — physically, socially/emotionally, and cognitively.

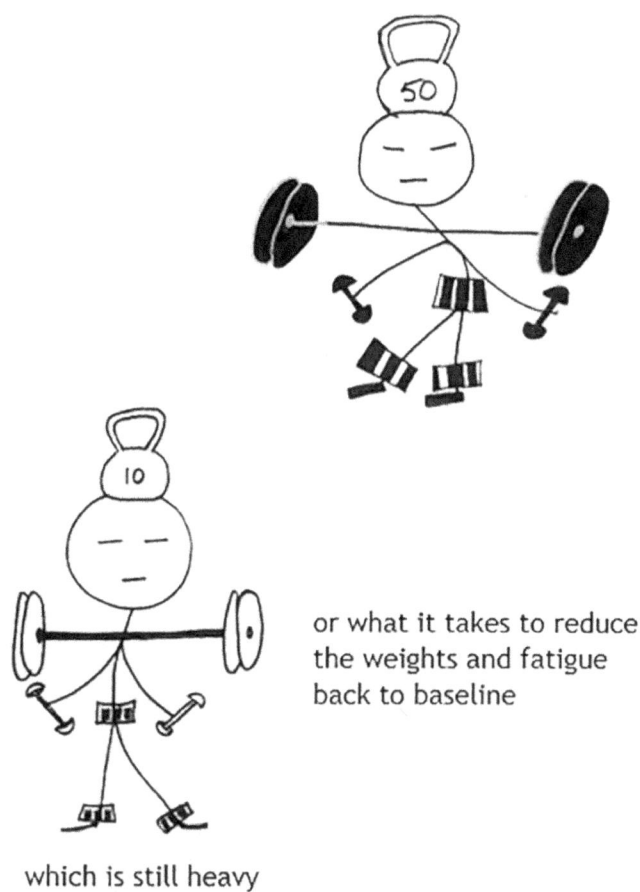

or what it takes to reduce the weights and fatigue back to baseline

which is still heavy

These three kinds of energy expenditures all burn the same amount.

It's draining, but I try to act normal.

If I act sick or try to explain myself, it's pretty hard for others to comprehend. I don't look like anything is wrong.

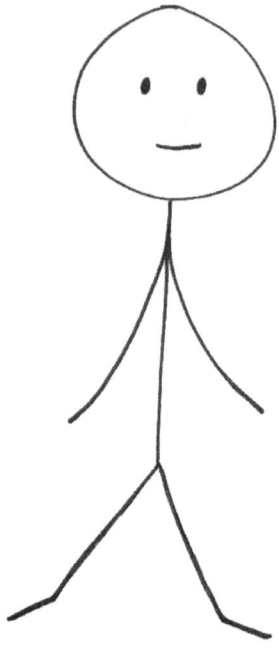

People got uncomfortable. I stopped trying to explain. I wrote this little book — it makes things easier for the people who are sincerely curious and for me.

When others judge, it hurts:

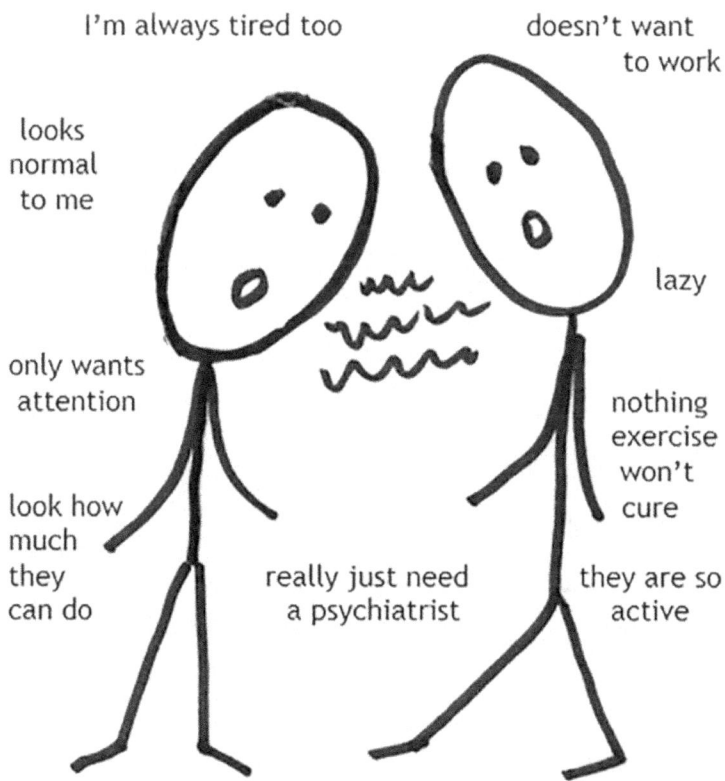

They have no idea what they are criticizing.

When I'm with you — you can't see the four symptoms I am never without.

- Weighted fatigue

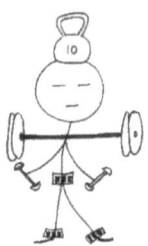

- Dizziness or a constant sense of motion

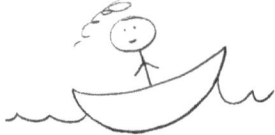

- Ringing in my ears

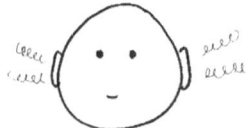

- Burning and tingling in my feet and legs

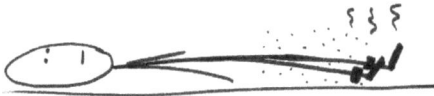

The others come and go, but the intensity of all are based on previous energy expenditure.

It is not "just being tired."
It is the sum total of many life factors.

You see this

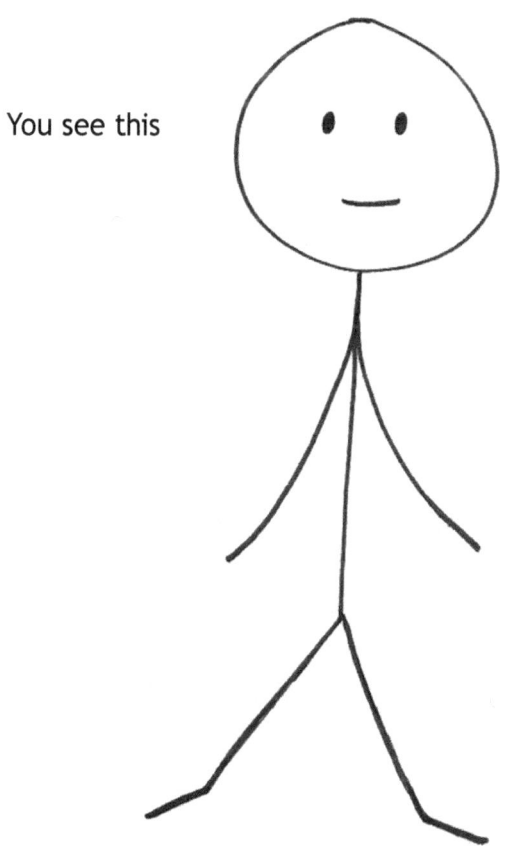

But there is so much you don't see.
I don't want sympathy, just understanding.

Don't shame me, don't judge me.

Anderson

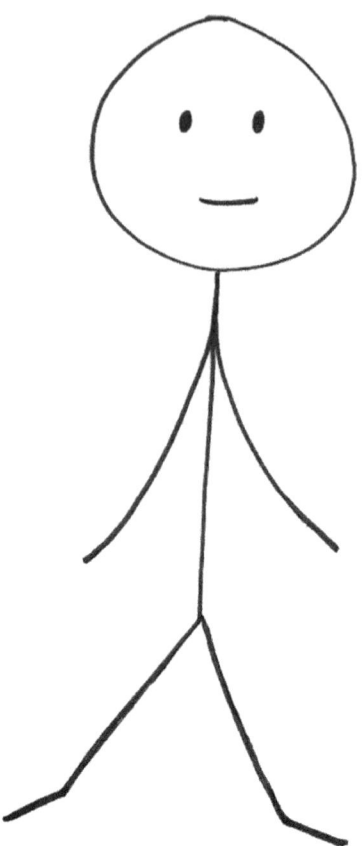

What you see is not how I feel

What can friends and loved ones do?

- Ask specifically what would help, even for a list of tasks to choose from.

- Choose a task(s) that is manageable for you and your schedule. Don't promise what you can't do.

- Text or email – don't phone, they may need time to answer.

- Set up an encouraging family or friends group chat to help them stay connected.

- Send a note of cheer or inspiration.

- Write about a funny experience or send a picture or short video (kids, pets, events, etc.).

- Don't always expect an answer.

- Learn about the illness, but don't give unsolicited advice (especially miracle cures).

"I wish they could feel what I feel."

I went way past my energy limit today. At 3:30 pm my head is filled with ear-splitting ringing. My feet and calves are tingling and burning; I feel tight bands squeezing my ankles. At the computer, I feel like I'm being tipped backward in my chair. My head drops back, I jerk it upright. I should be lying down, but needed to write this. I will pay for it tomorrow.

Then next morning, I get out of bed and walk down the hall. I feel like I'm on a boat rocking with short, choppy sideways waves. The rocking changes to long back and forth waves as I get coffee and sit down. A heavier weight than normal presses from my head down through my spine. There is pressure at the base of my skull, but the ringing of yesterday isn't as loud. The bands around my ankles have loosened. I sleep three times today; normally it's once or twice.

The intensity of my symptoms is proportionate to the energy I expend. Symptoms are mild when I ration energy, but they rage when I have overdone it.

I make choices. If there is a task that must be done, I do it knowing I will have to recover. Yet I am judged outwardly for the task — not the physical and emotional toll it takes on my body. Can anyone "see" what I am feeling? I wish they could feel what I feel.

About the Author

Anderson wrote this book as a simple visual tool to make clear that while appearing normal, living with Chronic Fatigue is a life-changing and controlling disease with a complex combination and fluctuation of symptoms that cannot be seen.

Adjusting to change, letting go of control, focusing on well-being, practicing yoga, and simply trusting and accepting what is has been a profound learning experience for Anderson.

www.ingramcontent.com/pod-product-compliance
Lightning Source LLC
LaVergne TN
LVHW021747060526
838200LV00052B/3529